DEFEATING THE SILENT KILLER

A COMPREHENSIVE GUIDE TO ENDING TUBERCULOSIS

ALEX USIFO

To the countless individuals, healthcare professionals, researchers, and advocates who have dedicated their lives to the fight against tuberculosis. Your unwavering commitment to eradicating this ancient scourge inspires us all.

To the survivors of tuberculosis, your courage and resilience shine as beacons of hope. Your stories remind us of the human spirit's capacity to overcome adversity.

To the memory of those who lost their lives to tuberculosis, may your legacy be a driving force in our collective pursuit of a tuberculosis-free world.

And to the global community, united in the battle against this silent threat, may our shared efforts bring us closer to a future where tuberculosis is no longer a burden on humanity.

This book is dedicated to each one of you, for your part in the ongoing struggle to defeat tuberculosis. Thank you for your unwavering dedication and belief in a healthier world for all.

CONTENTS

Introduction

Tuberculosis, often simply referred to as TB, has been a formidable adversary in the realm of infectious diseases for centuries. This book, "Tuberculosis Unveiled: Understanding, Managing, and Eradicating TB," delves into the complex world of tuberculosis, exploring its origins, impact, management, and global efforts to combat this persistent public health threat.

TB is a disease that has shaped societies, influenced cultures, and touched the lives of millions. It's a disease that knows no boundaries, affecting individuals from all walks of life and every corner of the globe. Understanding TB and the multifaceted approaches required to manage and ultimately eliminate it is not just a medical imperative; it's a moral one.

The purpose of this book is to provide a comprehensive resource that demystifies TB. We will journey through its history, gain insight into the science behind the disease, explore its social and psychological ramifications, and assess the tools and strategies available for diagnosis, treatment, and prevention. Moreover, we will examine the collective determination of the global community to eradicate TB from the face of the earth.

Each chapter is designed to be informative, engaging, and accessible, whether you're a healthcare professional, a patient, a caregiver, or someone simply seeking to better understand this ancient yet persistent disease.

Our exploration begins with the basics: an understanding of TB's origins, its transmission, and the various forms it can take within the human body. We will then move on to the critical aspects of diagnosis, treatment, and the challenges that healthcare providers and patients face along the way.

Lifestyle and nutrition are explored as integral elements of the recovery process, as well as the profound impact of TB on the psyche and social fabric. We delve into the support systems available for patients and how communities can collectively combat stigma and discrimination.

Prevention and control strategies come next, examining the power of vaccines, preventive therapy, and public health initiatives. We assess the global efforts to combat TB, from international goals to grassroots activism.

Finally, we peer into the future, exploring the exciting world of TB research, diagnostic innovations, and the quest for new drugs and vaccines. We also envision a world without TB and the road we must travel to achieve this audacious goal.

We hope that "Tuberculosis Unveiled" not only informs but also inspires. We invite you to embark on this enlightening journey through the realm of tuberculosis, a journey that begins with understanding, proceeds with effective management, and concludes with the eradication of this age-old adversary. Together, we can unveil the secrets of TB and work toward a healthier and TB-free world.

TB SYMPTOMS, DIAGNOSIS, AND TRANSMISSION

Tuberculosis (TB) is a complex and insidious disease that often hides in the shadows, making early diagnosis and treatment critical. In this chapter, we will explore the various aspects of TB, from its symptoms to diagnostic techniques and how it spreads.

Section 1: Recognizing TB Symptoms

TB is known for its diverse range of symptoms, which can manifest differently in each individual. Common symptoms include:

Persistent Cough: A cough that lasts for more than two weeks is one of the hallmark symptoms of pulmonary TB. It often produces sputum or blood.

Fever: Low-grade fever, often in the afternoon or evening, is a common sign of active TB infection.

Unexplained Weight Loss: TB can lead to unintentional weight loss and muscle wasting, which can be particularly concerning if accompanied by a decreased appetite.

Fatigue: Profound and unrelenting fatigue can be an early sign of active TB infection.

Night Sweats: Profuse sweating at night, leading to drenched bedclothes and sheets, is a typical symptom.

Chest Pain: Pain or discomfort in the chest, often when breathing or coughing, may occur in pulmonary TB.

Shortness of Breath: TB can lead to difficulty breathing, especially during physical activity.

It's essential to recognize these symptoms and seek medical attention if they persist. However, some individuals may have latent TB infection, where the bacteria are present but not causing symptoms. Early diagnosis can prevent the progression of latent TB to active disease.

Section 2: Diagnosis and Screening

TB Diagnosis: The diagnosis of TB involves several methods, including:

Sputum Tests: The examination of sputum samples for the presence of Mycobacterium tuberculosis, the bacterium causing TB.

Chest X-rays: Imaging to visualize abnormalities in the lungs, such as infiltrates or cavities.

Tuberculin Skin Test (TST): A skin test that detects a delayed-type hypersensitivity response to TB proteins.

Interferon-Gamma Release Assays (IGRAs): Blood tests that measure the immune response to TB proteins.

Bronchoscopy: An invasive procedure to collect lung samples for diagnosis.

Challenges in TB Diagnosis: TB diagnosis can be challenging due to several factors, including:

The slow growth of Mycobacterium tuberculosis in cultures.

Overlapping symptoms with other diseases.

The presence of drug-resistant TB strains that require specific tests for detection.

Preventive Measures: Healthcare providers play a vital role in early diagnosis by maintaining a high index of suspicion for TB, especially in high-risk populations. Prompt and accurate diagnosis is crucial to prevent further transmission.

Section 3: TB Transmission

TB spreads from person to person through the air when an infected individual expels infectious respiratory droplets. Key points regarding TB transmission include:

Human-to-Human Transmission: TB is primarily transmitted through close and prolonged contact with an infectious individual. Common scenarios include households, healthcare settings, and congregate settings like prisons.

Latent TB and Transmission: Individuals with latent TB infection are not infectious, as the bacteria are not actively replicating. However, if the latent infection progresses to active disease, transmission becomes possible.

Preventive Measures: Preventing TB transmission involves:

Identifying and isolating infectious individuals during their treatment.

Encouraging good respiratory hygiene, such as covering one's mouth when coughing.

Immunizing children with the Bacillus Calmette-Guérin (BCG) vaccine in regions with high TB prevalence.

Understanding the symptoms, diagnostic methods, and modes of transmission of TB is crucial for early detection and effective prevention, as discussed in this chapter. The next chapters will focus on the treatment, management, and prevention of TB, as well as the global efforts to combat this pervasive disease.

TB TREATMENT

Effective treatment of tuberculosis (TB) is paramount to curing the disease, preventing its spread, and ultimately saving lives. This chapter explores various facets of TB treatment, from the medications used to the strategies for managing the disease.

Section 1: TB Medications

The Armamentarium Against TB: TB treatment relies on a combination of antibiotics, primarily isoniazid, rifampin, pyrazinamide, and ethambutol. These medications target the Mycobacterium tuberculosis bacterium at different stages of its life cycle.

Drug-Resistant TB: Drug-resistant TB strains, including multidrug-resistant TB (MDR-TB) and extensively drug-resistant TB (XDR-TB), require more extensive and complex drug regimens. Treating drug-resistant TB is challenging, often involving second-line drugs with more side effects.

Drug Regimens for Different Forms of TB: TB treatment varies based on whether it is pulmonary or extrapulmonary TB, as well as the patient's overall health and drug susceptibility. Tailored treatment plans are essential.

Section 2: Standard TB Treatment Regimen

Directly Observed Treatment, Short-course (DOTS): DOTS is a standardized strategy recommended by the World Health Organization (WHO) for TB treatment. It includes:

Direct Observation: Healthcare workers or trained community members observe and document each dose of medication.

Treatment Regimens: Specific treatment regimens are provided based on the patient's age, weight, drug susceptibility, and type of TB.

Supervision and Support: Patients receive ongoing supervision and support to ensure adherence and monitor for side effects.

Success Stories and Challenges in DOTS Implementation: DOTS has been successful in treating TB patients worldwide, but it also faces challenges such as healthcare infrastructure limitations and funding gaps.

Section 3: Side Effects and Adverse Reactions

Managing Side Effects: TB medications can cause a range of side effects, including nausea, liver toxicity, vision changes, and peripheral neuropathy. Managing these side effects is vital to maintain patient adherence.

Monitoring Treatment Progress: Routine monitoring is necessary to assess the effectiveness of treatment and to identify any complications. This includes laboratory tests to check for the presence of the bacterium and the response to treatment.

Drug-Drug Interactions: Some TB medications may interact with other drugs a patient is taking, which can impact treatment effectiveness. Healthcare providers must be vigilant in managing these interactions.

Effective TB treatment not only cures the individual but also prevents the spread of the disease to others. While TB treatment can be challenging due to long treatment durations and potential side effects, adhering to the prescribed regimen is crucial for success.

In the following chapters, we will explore the critical role of lifestyle and nutrition in supporting TB patients, as well as the psychological and social aspects of living with TB. Additionally, we will delve into the prevention and control of TB, including vaccination and public health measures

Micronutrient Deficiencies: TB patients are at risk of deficiencies in specific vitamins and minerals, such as vitamin D, vitamin C, and zinc. Dietary supplementation or adjustments can address these deficiencies.

Section 2: Lifestyle Adjustments

Rest and Recovery: Adequate rest is crucial for TB patients. Fatigue is common, and patients should listen to their bodies, prioritizing sleep and recovery.

Exercise and Physical Activity: Light exercise can be beneficial for patients with TB. It improves lung function, overall fitness, and mental well-being. However, strenuous activities may need to be avoided, especially during active disease.

Stress Management: Stress can weaken the immune system, making it harder for the body to combat TB. Patients should employ stress-reduction techniques such as relaxation exercises and mindfulness.

Tobacco and Alcohol Cessation: Smoking and excessive alcohol consumption can exacerbate TB symptoms and hinder recovery. Quitting or reducing these habits is strongly advised.

Preventing Infections: TB patients should be cautious around individuals with infectious diseases, as their immune systems may be compromised.

Lifestyle and nutrition are integral components of TB management, complementing the medical treatment prescribed by healthcare providers. Ensuring that patients have access to a balanced diet and promoting a supportive living environment are crucial steps in the fight against TB.

The subsequent chapters will explore the psychological and social aspects of living with TB, the importance of social and psychological support, and the global initiatives aimed at controlling and ultimately eradicating this ancient disease.

SOCIAL AND PSYCHOLOGICAL SUPPORT

Living with tuberculosis (TB) can be physically and emotionally challenging. In this chapter, we delve into the social and psychological aspects of TB, its impact on patients, and the vital role of support systems in their journey to recovery.

Section 1: Psychosocial Impact of TB

Coping with the Diagnosis: The diagnosis of TB can bring a range of emotions, including fear, anxiety, and stigma. Patients may experience a sense of isolation and concern about transmitting the disease to loved ones.

Depression and Anxiety: The uncertainty surrounding TB, the lengthy treatment duration, and the potential side effects of medications can contribute to feelings of depression and anxiety. Recognizing and addressing these issues is crucial.

Stigma and Discrimination: TB is often associated with social stigma and discrimination. Patients may face rejection from friends, family, or community members. This discrimination can have a profound impact on their mental health.

Section 2: Social Support

The Role of Family and Friends: Family and friends can be a significant source of support for TB patients. Their understanding, empathy, and encouragement are invaluable.

Support Groups: Participating in TB support groups or networks can provide patients with an opportunity to share experiences, gain insights, and reduce feelings of isolation.

Counseling and Therapy: Professional counseling or therapy can help patients navigate the emotional challenges of living with TB, offering strategies to cope with stress, anxiety, and depression.

Patient Empowerment: Encouraging patients to be active participants in their care can help them feel more in control of their health. This empowerment can boost self-esteem and resilience.

Section 3: Combating Stigma and Discrimination

Education and Awareness: Raising public awareness about TB and dispelling misconceptions is crucial to combat stigma and discrimination.

Legal Protections: Many countries have legal protections in place to prevent discrimination against TB patients. Advocacy and awareness campaigns can ensure these protections are upheld.

Community Engagement: Engaging communities in TB education and support efforts can foster a more inclusive and understanding environment for patients.

Supporting the mental and emotional well-being of TB patients is integral to their recovery. Providing a supportive, non-discriminatory environment and access to mental health resources can significantly improve the patient's journey. In the subsequent chapters, we will explore preventive measures and global initiatives in the fight against TB, emphasizing the importance of a comprehensive approach to managing this disease.

PREVENTING TB

Preventing tuberculosis (TB) is a cornerstone of global efforts to control the disease and ultimately eliminate it. In this chapter, we will explore the strategies and measures in place to prevent TB at the individual, community, and societal levels.

Section 1: TB Prevention Strategies

Bacillus Calmette-Guérin (BCG) Vaccine: The BCG vaccine is used to prevent severe forms of TB, particularly in children. We will discuss its effectiveness, availability, and regions where it is administered.

Preventive Therapy for Latent TB Infection: Individuals with latent TB infection can receive preventive therapy to reduce the risk of developing active TB disease. We will explore the criteria for treatment and its effectiveness.

Airborne Infection Control: In healthcare settings, ensuring effective ventilation and infection control measures is essential to prevent the transmission of TB to healthcare workers and other patients.

Section 2: TB Control Programs

National TB Programs: Many countries have established National TB Programs to address the disease's burden. These programs focus on early detection, treatment, and monitoring of TB cases.

Directly Observed Treatment, Short-course (DOTS): We will further explore the DOTS strategy, which is endorsed by the World Health Organization (WHO) and has been instrumental in improving TB treatment outcomes worldwide.

Contact Tracing: Identifying and screening individuals who have been in close contact with TB patients is an important step in preventing further transmission.

Section 3: The Global Effort to Combat TB

The WHO's End TB Strategy: The World Health Organization's End TB Strategy sets global targets and outlines key interventions for reducing TB incidence, deaths, and catastrophic costs to households affected by TB.

International Initiatives: We will discuss international efforts to combat TB, including financial support, research initiatives, and partnerships with organizations such as the Global Fund to Fight AIDS, Tuberculosis, and Malaria.

Public Awareness Campaigns: Public awareness is a critical component of TB prevention. Initiatives to educate communities about TB, its symptoms, and how to access healthcare services are essential.

Research and Innovation: Ongoing research into TB diagnostics, drugs, and vaccines is vital to improving prevention efforts and treatment outcomes.

Preventing TB is a shared responsibility, involving individuals, healthcare systems, communities, and international organizations. Understanding the prevention strategies and being proactive in implementing them is essential in the fight against this persistent disease.

In the upcoming chapters, we will delve into the future of TB management, research and innovations, and the road to achieving the ambitious goal of a world free from TB.

TB IN SPECIAL POPULATIONS

Tuberculosis (TB) is a disease that can affect various population groups differently. In this chapter, we will explore how TB impacts specific populations, including children and individuals living with HIV, and the specialized considerations for managing TB in these groups.

Section 1: TB in Children

TB in Pediatric Patients: Children are a vulnerable population when it comes to TB. We will discuss the unique challenges in diagnosing and treating TB in children, who often present with atypical symptoms.

Preventive Measures for Children: Emphasizing the importance of TB prevention strategies, including BCG vaccination and preventive therapy, to protect children from TB infection.

Section 2: TB and HIV Co-Infection

The Intersection of TB and HIV: Individuals living with HIV are at a significantly higher risk of developing active TB. We will explore the challenges of managing TB in this population.

Co-Management of TB and HIV: The simultaneous treatment of TB and HIV requires a coordinated approach, often involving antiretroviral therapy (ART) and TB medications. We will discuss the strategies and challenges of co-management.

Preventive Measures for HIV-Positive Individuals: The importance of regular TB screening for individuals with HIV and the use of isoniazid preventive therapy to reduce the risk of TB.

Section 3: TB in Other Special Populations

TB in Pregnant Women: The unique considerations for diagnosing and treating TB in pregnant women and minimizing risks to both the mother and the unborn child.

TB in the Elderly: The challenges of diagnosing and treating TB in older adults, who may present with comorbidities and atypical symptoms.

TB in Congregate Settings: Managing TB in congregate settings such as prisons, homeless shelters, and long-term care facilities, where the risk of transmission is higher due to close living conditions.

TB in Migrants and Refugees: The importance of addressing TB in migrant and refugee populations, who may face additional barriers to healthcare access.

Understanding how TB affects special populations and tailoring prevention, diagnosis, and treatment to their unique needs is essential for effective management and control of the disease. In the following chapters, we will explore the future of TB management, including research and innovations, as well as the global efforts to combat TB and the path toward achieving a TB-free world.

THE FUTURE OF TB MANAGEMENT

The fight against tuberculosis (TB) continues to evolve with advances in research, technology, and healthcare systems. In this chapter, we will explore the future of TB management, including research and innovations that hold promise for improving prevention, diagnosis, treatment, and ultimately, eradicating the disease.

Section 1: Research and Innovations

New Diagnostic Technologies: Emerging diagnostic tools, such as molecular diagnostics and point-of-care tests, promise quicker and more accurate TB diagnosis, reducing the time to initiate treatment.

New Drug Development: Ongoing research is focused on developing novel TB drugs that are more effective, less toxic, and have shorter treatment durations. This includes research into the treatment of drug-resistant TB.

Vaccines: Research continues to develop more effective TB vaccines that can provide better protection against the disease, including for adults.

Treatment Shortening: Shorter, more manageable treatment regimens for TB are being explored, which could improve patient adherence and outcomes.

Section 2: The Road to Eradication

The Global Goal: The global goal of eradicating TB is ambitious, and we will explore the progress and challenges faced in achieving this objective.

Research into Transmission: Understanding the transmission dynamics of TB is crucial to effectively interrupting the spread of the disease.

Active Case Finding: Proactive efforts to find and treat individuals with TB, especially in high-risk populations, can accelerate the reduction of TB incidence.

Comprehensive Care: Providing comprehensive care, including psychosocial support, nutritional support, and preventive therapy, is integral to achieving successful TB management.

Section 3: The Role of Community Engagement

Community Participation: Engaging communities in TB awareness and support efforts can reduce stigma, improve early case detection, and promote treatment adherence.

Patient Advocacy: Empowering patients and those affected by TB to advocate for their needs and access to quality care is a driving force for change.

Multi-Sectoral Collaboration: Collaboration between healthcare, government, and non-governmental organizations is critical for effective TB management and control.

The future of TB management is marked by innovation, research, and a concerted effort to overcome the challenges of TB prevention, diagnosis, and treatment. Achieving a world free from TB is an audacious goal, but with continued dedication to research, global collaboration, and community engagement, it is an achievable one.

In the following chapters, we will discuss the importance of public awareness, advocacy, and global initiatives aimed at combating TB on a larger scale

CONCLUSION

Tuberculosis, a disease that has plagued humanity for centuries, remains a global challenge. However, significant progress has been made in the understanding, management, and prevention of tuberculosis (TB). This journey through the chapters of this book, "Tuberculosis Unveiled: Understanding, Managing, and Eradicating TB," has provided insights into the various facets of TB, from its symptoms and diagnosis to treatment, lifestyle and nutrition, social and psychological support, prevention, and the future of TB management.

Recognizing the symptoms of TB and seeking prompt diagnosis are critical steps in controlling the disease. Through advancements in diagnostic tools and research into more accurate and rapid testing, the ability to identify and treat TB cases has improved significantly. The critical role of directly observed treatment (DOTS) in ensuring patient adherence to treatment regimens has been emphasized.

Lifestyle modifications and proper nutrition have been highlighted as essential elements of recovery. Adequate rest, exercise, stress management, and a balanced diet are instrumental in supporting the body's healing process. Addressing the psychosocial impact of TB, including depression, anxiety, and the stigma associated with the disease, is fundamental to improving the overall well-being of TB patients.

Prevention strategies, including vaccination and preventive therapy, are central to reducing the global burden of TB. The importance of national TB programs and the World Health Organization's End TB Strategy has been underscored in the fight against the disease. The future of TB management is marked by research and innovations, such as new diagnostic technologies, more effective drugs, and the quest for a better TB vaccine.

The path to TB eradication requires active case finding, community engagement, and multi-sectoral collaboration. It is a collective effort involving healthcare providers, governments, non-governmental organizations, and, most importantly, individuals and communities.

The role of patient advocacy, community support, and public awareness campaigns cannot be underestimated in achieving a world free from TB.

In conclusion, TB is a persistent global health challenge, but it can be overcome with continued dedication, research, and a comprehensive approach to management and prevention. The journey to a TB-free world is ambitious, but it is a journey worth embarking on to save lives, reduce suffering, and create a healthier and more equitable world for all. Together, we can unveil the secrets of TB and work toward a brighter, TB-free future.

Certainly, here are some definitions of medical terms related to tuberculosis (TB):

Tuberculosis (TB): A bacterial infection caused by Mycobacterium tuberculosis, primarily affecting the lungs but potentially spreading to other parts of the body.

Mycobacterium tuberculosis: The bacterium responsible for causing TB. It has a thick, waxy cell wall that makes it difficult to treat with many antibiotics.

Pulmonary TB: TB that primarily affects the lungs, leading to symptoms like cough, chest pain, and difficulty breathing.

Extrapulmonary TB: TB that affects parts of the body other than the lungs, such as the bones, lymph nodes, or kidneys.

Latent TB Infection (LTBI): A condition in which an individual is infected with the TB bacterium but does not show symptoms of the disease and is not contagious. However, the bacteria can become active later if the immune system weakens.

Active TB Disease: When TB bacteria become active and cause symptoms, such as fever, cough, and weight loss. Active TB is contagious.

Tuberculin Skin Test (TST): A test that involves injecting a small amount of purified protein derivative (PPD) under the skin to assess a person's response to TB proteins. It is used to detect TB infection but cannot distinguish between latent and active TB.

Interferon-Gamma Release Assay (IGRA): A blood test that detects the presence of an immune response to TB-specific antigens. IGRA is used to diagnose TB infection, similar to the tuberculin skin test.

Multidrug-Resistant TB (MDR-TB): TB that is resistant to at least two of the most potent first-line anti-TB drugs, isoniazid and rifampin.

Extensively Drug-Resistant TB (XDR-TB): A severe form of drug-resistant TB that is resistant to not only isoniazid and rifampin but also to additional second-line drugs, making it more challenging to treat.

Directly Observed Treatment, Short-course (DOTS): A standardized approach to TB treatment that involves direct observation of patients taking their medication. It is recommended by the World Health Organization to ensure treatment adherence.

Bacillus Calmette-Guérin (BCG) Vaccine: A vaccine that provides partial protection against severe forms of TB, primarily in children. It is often administered in regions with a high prevalence of TB.

Preventive Therapy: The use of medication, such as isoniazid, to prevent individuals with latent TB infection from developing active TB disease.

Sputum Test: A diagnostic test that involves examining a sample of a patient's sputum (mucus coughed up from the lower airways) for the presence of TB bacteria.

Chest X-ray: A medical imaging test that provides images of the lungs and chest to identify abnormalities, such as TB-related lung infiltrates or cavities.

Contact Tracing: The process of identifying and screening individuals who have been in close contact with a confirmed TB patient to determine if they have been infected.

Isoniazid (INH): A first-line anti-TB medication used to treat TB infection and disease.

Rifampin: Another first-line anti-TB drug that is used in combination with other medications to treat TB.

Multidrug Therapy: A treatment approach for TB that combines several anti-TB drugs to prevent the development of drug resistance.

Bronchoscopy: An invasive medical procedure in which a thin, flexible tube is inserted into the airways to collect samples from the lungs for diagnosis.

These definitions provide an overview of key medical terms related to tuberculosis and its diagnosis and treatment.

ABOUT THE AUTHOR

ALEX USIFO

Dr. Alex Usifo is a highly respected researcher with over two decades of experience in the field of medicine. I have made significant contributions to the medical field through her clinical work, research, and her role in mentoring the next generation of medical professionals. I have published numerous articles in reputable medical journals and have been at the forefront of groundbreaking research in areas such as cardiovascular medicine and preventive healthcare.

My motivation as an author of medical books is to bridge the gap between medical knowledge and patient understanding. She is deeply committed to making complex medical concepts accessible to the general public and to healthcare professionals seeking to expand their knowledge.

This book covers a wide range of medical topics, from comprehensive guides on specific medical conditions and their treatments to books focusing on wellness, nutrition, and lifestyle choices for maintaining optimal health. My works provide valuable insights for patients, caregivers, and healthcare practitioners alike. As a medical author, my work serves as a valuable resource for those seeking to better understand medical conditions, treatment options, and the importance of maintaining good health. Her dedication to improving healthcare literacy and her contributions to medical literature have positively impacted countless lives.